ESCAPE THAT FAT

HOW TO LOSE WEIGHT FAST AND FOREVER

BY

TINA JOHNSON

INTRODUCTION

Wouldn't it be great if we all knew what lay in our future, if we could just see what was around the next corner? Then if we knew a problem was about to come up, we could change things to avoid the problem, or be prepared for when it came.

While it's impossible to know all our future, and maybe that's a good thing, we can prepare ourselves better for what's up ahead...even in weight loss. But before we look to see if you're heading for a weight loss disaster, let's take a moment to look at what a mistake really means.

The Meaning of Mistakes

Nobody likes making mistakes, myself included. It's frustrating when something doesn't turn out the way we wanted it to. But while making mistakes can sometimes be painful, they are there to teach us a lesson. Or to put it differently if we substituted the word "mistake" with the word "feedback" we'd tend to look at mistakes in a different light.

The thing is we tend to take mistakes very personally. We fail at something like losing weight then we start to think it's because we're useless, lazy or different from everyone else, and we'll never succeed. But is that fair or shouldn't we look for the "feedback" for our answers?

An important thing to keep in mind is that when fail or make a mistake, it's an event rather than a person.

For example if you were making a cake and it turned out wrongly, does that mean you're in some way a lesser person? Or does it mean that you didn't follow the instructions of the recipe to the letter. Because if you did wouldn't you get the same results as everyone else?

The same is true for weight loss.

Are You Heading For A Weight Loss Disaster?

So are you heading for a disaster with your new attempt at losing weight? Not sure? Then I want you to think back to the last time you tried to diet unsuccessfully? How do you think it all went wrong?

You probably have some ideas, go grab a pen and write down where you think you went wrong with your last dieting attempt. If you're honest with yourself, you probably know already what happened.

But here are some possible reasons...

Making the Wrong Food Choices? - Although you knew you needed to change your eating habits, you did nothing about it?

Dieting With the Wrong People? - While our best friends might have our best wishes at heart are they in the best position to give dieting or exercise advice, or would it be better to talk to a professional.

Giving Up Too Soon? - While we all live in an instant gratification society, unfortunately weight loss takes time. That weight didn't appear overnight and it's not going to disappear in the same space of time.

Doing the Wrong Exercise Routine? – Did you try to do an exercise routine that you knew from the start, was impossible to stick to? For example if you've never been one to exercise much, could you honestly expect to stick to a exercise routine that only a "Navy Seal" could do?

So, have you got your list made out?

Did you know you've just done something that 99% of people who want to lose weight don't do?

You've now got a list of where you've gone wrong, and what mistakes you've made in the past. Now if you work on correcting these things you'll get better results. If you think about it, how crazy is it to make the same mistakes over and over again and expect different results?

Now that you have you your list I want you to pick 2 that you think are the biggest mistakes you've made. Then read on how the 80/20 rule can make weight loss a lot easier...

HOW THE 80-20 RULE MAKES FOR EASIER WEIGHT LOSS

For those of you not familiar with the 80 - 20 rules I'll explain it here. The 80/20 rule is a universal rule that applies to every topic of life, from business, relationships to health.

To break it down to its very basics, it means that 20% of effort gives you 80% of your results, and 80% of your effort only gives you 20% of your results.

If we take someone running a store as an example, they may find that 20% of your products give them 80% of their profits. While the other 80% brings in only 20% of their profits.

So how can you use this rule in your favour?

20% Of Bad Habits Cause 80% of Your Problems - Make a list of your bad eating habits, you'll probably notice that there are 1-2 habits that you do again and again that are causing all your weight problems. You may notice that snacking in front of the TV is a big mistake you make. Then simply change that habit and you will notice a big difference in your weight loss

Reduce Your Plate Size by 20% - Try to find plates that are 20% smaller than the ones you normally use. It might sound like a small thing to do but it can bring about big results.

80% Of Gym Time Is Wasted Time - If you're looking to reduce time and burn more calories focus more on building muscle mass than on cardio work. Although cardio has its place, the faster and more permanent way to boost your metabolism is to build more muscle mass.

80% Of Car Journey are Probably Wasted Journeys - While we all need cars to get about, if you look at how many journeys you make each day, you may see that you don't need to do all of them in a car. If you've gotten into the habit of jumping into the car for that 2 minute drive to the local store, why not leave the car in the driveway and use a bike or walk instead?

80% Of Watching TV Is Wasted Time – Many people complain that they never have time to exercise, but like everyone else we only have 24 hours. So, how are you spending yours? You may be surprised how much time in your day is wasted watching TV. Possibly watching programs you don't like, or channel surfing out of habit. If you think about it, t there are really only a core selection of programs that we really watch (about 20%). So why not stick to only that, and forget the others (80%). You now have this extra time to jump on a cycling machine or treadmill at home or just simply go out for a walk.

While the 80/20 rule isn't an exact science that everything falls into exactly 80% and 20%. You will find that even changing small things on one side can make huge differences on the other side.

So why not use it in your favour instead of against you!

Now if you only focused on just correcting 2 mistakes in your list you'd find weight loss a lot easier and more importantly permanent .

The Golden Rules of Successful Weight Loss.

Here's what I think are the 9 golden rules for *permanent* weight loss...

1 - Weight Loss Success Leaves Clues - You'd never ask your broke neighbour for financial advice, so why ask someone who hasn't had any success losing weight for advice? Find someone who's lost weight successfully and KEPT it off long

2 - You Get Out What You Put In - One of the major rules of life is the law of cause and effect or action and reaction. To break it down to its basics, you get out what you put in. If you're not happy with your results simply put more effort in.

3 - Become A Different Person - Following on from tip 2, ask yourself what do thin people do that I don't do...then do it. The situation you're in is because of the person you are and the habits you have, so it wouldn't it make sense that you need to change, to get different results?

4 - Do Something You Love - If going to the gym or running 5 miles every morning isn't for you, don't do it. Find something you love and stick with that whether it's walking, playing tennis, basketball, whatever...you'll be more inclined to stick to it and burn fat doing something you love.

5 - Weight Loss Takes Time - If you think about we all don't put on weight overnight and its not going to disappear overnight. You might want instant results, but it only brings temporary results. So what if it takes you 2 years to lose 60 pounds, 2 years may sound like a lot of time but those 2 years will pass anyway, so why not use them to bring you closer to your goal?

6 - You're In Charge of Your Life - A lot of people have a lottery mentality. When they win the lottery their life will change. But, I'm sorry to bust any bubbles here, but it may never happen. The only one in charge of your life is YOU. You can wait all your life hoping that someone is going to rescue you from your weight problem, but it's not going to happen. Get behind the steering wheel of your life and steer it where you want it to go!

7 - Become A Goal Setter - The most successful people in life are those that have a goal or target. They then work towards it, to bring their current situation closer to their dream situation. Think about what you want to achieve and write it down. Now you know where you want to be rather than aimlessly losing one or two pounds and not having any direction.

8 - Do Something Every Day towards Your Goal - If you finish everyday having done something towards your goal you'll go to bed happy. I know from personal experience how satisfied I am from looking over the list of things I've done that day, knowing that its bringing me closer to my goal. Try it and you'll wonder why you've never used this technique before.

9 – Finally, A Failures Not A Failure - We all have this fear of failure. We don't do things in case we fail, but it's not failure its feedback! Change your thinking of failure from "I did it and it didn't work" to "It didn't work, so what do I need to change to get a better result next time?" Learn from your failures and move on, don't make the same mistakes over and over again without learning the lesson

Let's take a look at one why you can turn failure around...

MAKING A WEIGHT LOSS GOAL

Making goals isn't something the majority of us do nowadays, we go through life from day to day and wonder why things never change. Why is that? Could it be that we don't have any goals to direct our lives to where we want to be?

If you've ever gone on a road trip or holiday, you'll know how important it is to plan out your trip. You probably worked out what clothes you'd wear, documents you needed to bring, checked your car for gas, etc. You know that having all these details sorted and planned out in advance, would make your holiday run a whole lot smoother and leave nothing to chance.

You'd never think of leaving anything to chance if your holiday was that important would you? But why is it that 99 out of 100 of us, don't use this type of thinking when it comes to losing weight?

We start a diet on a Monday morning with a vague idea of what weight we'd like to lose and maybe how to get there, and that's it. But is vague good enough? Unfortunately not, vague plans always bring about vague results.

Let's take a look at your last diet, did you have a vague idea of getting slimmer but nothing concrete to aim for? If I were to ask you, when you'd know when you'd reached your goal would you be able to tell me? Probably not, but if losing weight was really important and at the forefront of your mind, wouldn't it make sense not to leave anything to chance. Wouldn't it be wise to plan out what you'd like to happen?

You'd never find an archer or sharp shooter, firing off shots blindly in all directions praying to hit the bull's-eye. Of course not, and why would you. They've got a target or bull eye to aim for and they keep trying until they hit it. Having a weight loss goal gives you something concrete to work towards, and gives you something to measure your progress by. But what if you've never made a weight loss goal before how would you do it?

Here are 7 steps to help you create a goal that can propel you on to that slimmer and healthier version of you....

Step 1 - Grab A Pen And Paper.

This is your *first big step* towards a slimmer you, so don't skip it. Doing this proves to the inner you that you're serious about this new commitment to yourself. I'm a big believer in writing things down as it helps to make you think about what you're doing.

Step 2 - What Are Your 5 Greatest Achievement's.

This tip might sound a bit strange but stick with me here. Have you ever won an award for anything, can you do something that others find difficult?

Make a list of 5 things that have happened in your life that you're proud of. These things may have happened this year, or times gone by, it doesn't matter. Just pick five things that make you feel proud about yourself.

The idea behind this tip is that it makes you aware that even though you have a weight problem you're not a failure. This may be a part of life that isn't working out but "Hey look at all you've achieved in other areas of your life!"

Step 3 - How Much Weight Do You Want To Lose?

Now write down how much weight you'd like to lose this year. (Be realistic you can't expect to lose 40 pounds in 3 weeks) pick a figure that's both achievable and also a little out of your reach. A good guide to healthy weight loss is one pound per week. You may easily beat this weekly target, but one pound a week is a good guideline to follow.

Step 4 - Why Do You Want To Lose Weight?

It may be obvious but each of you but each of us has our own unique reason for losing weight. What's yours...? Is it to prove to others that you're not a loser? Is it because you want better health? Is it because you're fed up buying larger clothes? Is it because you want to make your ex- partner jealous?

Now I want you to think, "WHY" do I want to lose weight? It's probably going to be different for everyone, so I can't give you an exact answer this is going to be your WHY. This is one of the most important steps you can take, if you have a big enough "WHY" you can do anything. Some mothers have been known to lift cars off their children because they had a big enough "WHY".

So, what's yours? Find the strongest reason that makes you want to lose weight. It may take a little time so think a little on it, but when you find a really strong "why" it can carry you through the tough days when you feel like giving up. Remember this has to be your reason, so don't write down because a friend or spouse wants you to lose weight. This won't keep you going, it's got to be *your* reason "WHY".

Step 5 - How Do I Need To Change As A Person?

What kind of person do you need to become to achieve this goal? You've probably heard the old saying "If you keep doing what you've always done you always get the same results". So ask yourself, if you continue to act the same way, every day, can you honestly expect things to change? But the opposite is also true, if you change those old actions with new ones, your results would also have to change!

So what do YOU have to change as a person to get where you want to go? Does it mean you need to get out of your comfort zone and go to a gym? Does it mean buying some new cookery books and learning to cook good natural food, rather than living on convenience foods full of fat and other nasties? Does it mean avoiding late night TV so you can get up early to prepare your daily meals, or get in some exercise?

Now write down 2 - 3 ways you need to change as a person. Of course you could write down more but you'd probably get overwhelmed and not put them into action. It's best to start small and work from there, you can always add more along the way.

You Should Now Have A List Of 4 Things

1. - 5 Things that you're proud of achieving.

2. - How much weight you want to lose

3. - "WHY" you want to lose weight

4. - 2 -3 Changes that will bring you closer to the person you need to become.

Now keep this list with you at all times, where you can refer to it again and again. Put it on the fridge, beside your bathroom mirror or anywhere you'll see it over and over again.

This is your map/checklist of where you want to be headed this year. As the next couple of week's go by, every day look over your list again and ask yourself "Was I faithful to what I wrote here?" Did I do all this week that I could to bring me closer to my goal? Because one things for sure if it's not bringing you closer to your goal, it's taking you further away from it.

How Weight Loss Goals Can Go Wrong.

While having a weight loss goal can be great, they can go wrong and for a number of reasons. When these things happen, it can knock your confidence and make the idea of setting any new weight loss goals in the future, very slim if not at all.

Here are 5 reasons your goal setting may fail...

Reason 1 - You May Have Set Your Weight Loss Goal Too High - When you set a goal that seems unreachable, you can give up before you even try. Set realistic goals that can seem more achievable, rather than focusing on the 40 pounds you need to lose, break it down to a smaller amount, like focusing on losing 5 pounds first and then build on that.

Reason 2 - Your Weight Loss Goals May Be Set Too Low - The opposite is also true if you focus on too small a weight loss goal, you may feel no challenge or benefit in achieving the goal. Remember always set goals that are challenging enough to be worth the effort, but not out of reach.

Reason 3 - Your Weight Loss Goal Is Too Vague - Is it 20 or 30 pounds you're looking to lose? If your achievement can't be measured, you can't see if you're reaching your goal or not. Know exactly how much you want to lose and aim for that figure only. If after that you need to lose more weight pick another target weight loss to hit.

Reason 4 - Weight Loss Goals Aren't Celebrated - If you aren't celebrating the achievement of reaching your goal (even a small one) what's the point of setting it in the first place? When you achieve your weight loss goal, go out and celebrate it, buy some new clothes, have a massage, a new hair style. But whatever you pick, stay away from food as a treat, you're only undoing your hard work.

Reason 5 - Having Too Many Goals - Having more than just one goal can be distracting and can complicate things and make you feel overwhelmed. Pick one goal and see it through to the end. Remember that you deserve time to relax and enjoy being alive, and not just solely focused on your goals and achievements.

When goal setting does go wrong, not only are the benefits of goal setting lost, but the whole process of having weight loss goals can seem a total waste of time. But by avoiding these problems, and setting your weight loss goals effectively, you can achieve and maintain a strong forward leap into your future slimmer you.

Now let's take a look at how to double your weight loss, without doing any exercise...

HOW TO DOUBLE YOUR WEIGHT LOSS EFFORTS WITHOUT EXERCISE

Wouldn't it be great if you could increase your weight loss results, even without exercise? It probably sounds too good to be true, but believe it or not, you can do this by simply using a food diary.

So, what is a food diary? A food diary is simply a day to day diary where you record everything you've eaten each day.

The advantages of using a food diary are that it...

• Helps stop unconscious eating. Because you can see what food you've eaten as it's all written down in black and white.

• Helps you to see what your bad eating habits are, and what you've been snacking on.

• Can make you think twice before eating junk food.

• May shock you into how much you really eat in your day.

That last point is one that a lot of TV dieting shows use to shock their overweight contestants. When they see how much food they consume on a daily basis (on table in front of them) it's usually enough to make them see that they need to turn things around. Often this alone is a wakeup call that they need to make a change to their lifestyle, and make them want to lose weight.

Proof That a Food Diary Does Have Benefits

In a study published in the American Journal of Preventive Medicine, people who kept a food diary lost an average 13 pounds more than people who didn't. The conclusion the researchers came to was that having and using a food diary, helped people to pick up on bad eating habits or behaviors that they weren't aware of. For example the simple habit of eating some cookies every time you sit in front of the TV can quickly add up the pounds. But this habit may have become so ingrained in your day to day life, that you mightn't notice it.

But Is A Food Diary Right For You?

If a food diary and recording your eating habits sounds like the thing you need, there are some things you need to keep in mind. Like most ways of losing weight, it all depends on you putting in some effort, like exercise equipment, if it's never used you'll never get the benefits. This is the same with a food diary, if it's never filled in, you'll never see the benefits. Honesty is a big part of having and keeping a food diary, if you pick and choose what goes in your food diary, you'll never get the results you're looking for.

But if you feel that this may be your downfall, ask someone you trust to keep a close eye on you and record your eating habits for you. It won't work as well as doing it yourself, but it's better than doing nothing.

How to Create a Food Diary

There are various way of keeping track of your food in a diary, either on an online website or offline in a simple note pad. I believe the second option is best and the easiest to do, the reason for this is that there can be a time delay between what you've eaten and when you write things down on a website. This can lead to leaving things out, and not writing everything down properly, which defeats the purpose.

So, when you've got a notepad in hand. Here are the 5 main points to jot down in your food diary...

1 – What Foods Have You Eaten and How Much? – This probably sounds obvious but by recording the foods you've eaten, you'll become more aware of what you've put in your mouth. It's like the equivalent of those diet shows, which show a contestant how much food they've eaten in a week. Remember, just because it disappeared in your mouth, doesn't mean it didn't exist. This alone could be a huge wake up call for you.

2 – Where Were You Eating? – Were you eating sitting down in front of the TV, at the kitchen table, at a restaurant? By recording where you were, you may notice a trend. Do you eat more when you're at home or eating out? Do you find yourself eating more in front of the TV? If you notice that some places or areas cause you to eat more, you can now avoid them and eat elsewhere.

3 – Who Were You Eating With? – Was it your best friend, or was it with your family, or were you eating alone? Like the last tip you'll start to notice a trend, if you find you eat more on your own, then try to eat in the company of others.

4 – What Time Did You Eat At? – Are you a midnight feaster or do you eat more at different times of the day? By recording the times you eat at, you can do more about this problem. It may lead you to stop eating after 7pm, or eat more in the earlier parts of the day when you've a better chance of burning it off.

5 – What Snacks Did You Eat during the Day – Like tip 1 there's no point in just recording meals and not recording your snacking? You might not have a problem with food, but snacking could be your downfall. Record what snacks you've eaten and how much. If you find snacking is a problem for you, either don't shop for these products, so they won't be in your house anymore OR buy the small snack version, and stick to eating only one, (remember just because it's smaller, doesn't mean you can get carried away eating lots of them).

NOTE - Remember a food diary will only work if you're honest and put everything (and I mean everything down), otherwise you're only fooling yourself, and you'll never get to the root of your weight problem.

Now that we've got the basics of properly recording your eating habits, let's take a look at how to turbo charge your weight loss motivation....

HOW TO FIRE UP YOUR MOTIVATION FOR WEIGHT LOSS

Being motivated and sticking to your weight loss plan can be hard, and there will be days when the scales don't move and you feel like throwing in the towel. So what can you do?

Here are 11 tips to start that motivation fire going again...

1 - Take It One Day at a Time - Even the longest journey or change in lifestyle all begins with a single step. While these small steps might not seem much, but if they're repeated over and over again momentum will start to build up. Take the example of pushing a car, the first couple of pushes are the hardest but once the wheels are turning, it takes less effort to keep the pace up. Just promise yourself that you're ONLY going to train just today, then say this to yourself the next day and the next day.

2 - Does Your Goal Excite You - Does losing weight excite you or are you just going through the motions? If a goal doesn't excite you, you'll never give it your full attention. Grab a pen and paper and write a list of what this weight loss will do you for you. Make a list of about 10-20 things that will change because you've lost that weight. Reading through this list when you've finished, should make you feel better about yourself and your goal.

3 - Visualize Your Success - If you haven't been successful how you can get that feeling of accomplishment, easy visualize! Some people say they have a problem with visualizing but we all do it. If I said what you would do if you won the lottery, I bet you'd have dozens of images flash through your mind. Now take that same power and picture how you'll feel and look in that slimmer future. If you're still having problems take your list from tip 2 and read through it for help, those answers should help put some great images in your mind.

4 - Get in a Team - While it's sometimes easy to get inspired for a short while, for longer periods sometimes we need others to give us that added kick up the pants. Try to find like-minded people who want to make a change in their lives and use them to inspire you. If you can't find anyone close by that you can rely on, or support from, why not use the internet and weight loss forums or help. Or if this isn't for you, why not look in books or weight loss magazines for inspirational stories that help lift you up. Another great place that's overlooked is YouTube.com, there you can find hundreds of great motivational and inspiring stories.

5 - Hold Back - It can be easy to throw yourself "Gung-ho" into your fitness at the beginning, but slowly over time you burn out and motivation fizzles away. So why not hold that motivation in check, if you feel that you could exercise for an hour why not cut back 25%, and exercise for three quarters of an hour. This way you know you've still got more in the tank for the next time, when maybe you'll give it a little bit more. This way you're going to increase in intensity as time goes on rather than do the opposite.

6 - Sleep More - Lack of sleep can take the zip out of anyone, so try to get your daily amount, then you'll be mentally fit and prepared for what's ahead.

7 - Organize Your Space - If you've got clothes thrown over the exercise bike and you constantly have to look for exercise clothes/equipment you need a declutter. Clear out a space that's solely yours for exercising. If you want you can also put some posters/motivation images around that you can look at as you work out. In short, make your exercise space a happy place that you look forward to visiting.

8 - Set Goals and Deadlines - Having a target or goal can be a great way to inspire yourself. Pick something small that you want to achieve like losing those first 5 pounds! Now go out and get it and don't stop until you've achieved it, then move on to the next goal. Unfinished goals can be a drain and kill motivation, but build on those small goals and you'll start to feel more positive that you can do it.

9 - Use Music - Music can be a great motivator when you're down. You could be in the worst mental state of your life but if your favorite song came on, you'd feel better in an instant. Burn a CD or load up your mp3 player with all those favorite tunes that make you want to get up and go.

10 - Get Outside - There's something magical that a bit of fresh air and change of scenery can do for us. If you're not feeling like exercising, just take a short walk to clear your mind and get the blood flowing. After 5- 10 minutes, don't be surprised if like "Forest Gump" you want to keep on going running and running.

11 - Use Past Failures to Succeed – Are you one of those people who hates being told what to do, does it make you want to do the opposite? Why not use this to power up your weight loss, call up all those old images of past failures or people telling you you'll never succeed, and use it against them. Think to yourself "I'll show them I can do it"...and then go out and do it!

Committing to your dreams takes hard work, but knowing how to motivate yourself can help you keep your eye on the prize. But as the saying goes, everything starts from your mind and the most powerful mind is a positive one. There will always be that little voice that says "You can't do it" but to counteract this, you can use visualization to build a positive image of what you want. Picture all that losing weight would mean to you, the comments from friends, shopping for new clothes etc. Build it all up in your mind like being at the movies and you should notice a more positive feeling in about yourself.

An interesting thing to remember is that as your mind as ability to change how your body feels the opposite is also true. For example if you're in a bad mood, if you put on a smile (even if it's a forced one), you'll notice that after some time your mood lightens. So, if you can't get your mind in gear, use your body instead. Make a fist and pound it in your opposite hand repeatedly, while making positive statements to yourself, "Yes, I can do this"..."I love to exercise"...or whatever else gets your blood up and pumping.

If you still can't get your mind in the right state, crank up the volume to your favorite song or use the sound track from your favorite inspiring movie. Take the "Rocky" theme as an example, who wouldn't want to get up and get moving after listening to that inspiring sound track.

Keeping Track Of Your Goals Can Also Improve Motivation.

What can be more inspiring than having a goal or target that you're aiming for? Setting goals is the one of the first steps in motivating yourself. Write down your goals in detail and write down how much time you want to achieve them. Now any small step you take toward your goals feeds your motivation. A major mistake that many people make is that they have the goals set, in their "mind" rather than written down. If you note down all your goals on paper along with the actions you need to take on a daily basis, you'll be more inclined to follow through.

Use Rewards To Motivate Yourself.

Rewards are a great motivator; take a 9 -5 job as an example. Employers have long known that a bonus to improve productivity always helps to motivate their staff. They still mightn't like their job but that bonus at the end of the project can make it all worthwhile. If you've got kids you'll know how great this technique works. If they behave themselves properly they get a treat for their good work. So why not use it on yourself as well, make a goal of how many days in a row you'll train, then when you reach it, and treat yourself for your great work. It doesn't have to be food, why not buy a new pair of trainers or a new tracksuit to show off that new figure?

Using the Pain/Pleasure Principle to Increase Motivation.

We all go through life using this principle, we do the things we love (that bring us pleasure) and avoid all those other nasty's that bring us pain. Food and the lack of exercise has given you great pleasure (that's why weight gain was easy) but it's also causing you discomfort. If it wasn't, you wouldn't want to lose that extra weight.

So why not build up the pain side of the argument, and get motivated by it. Get really uncomfortable with where you are in this present moment of your life and use it to power yourself along. What do you really hate about being fat and out of shape? Make a list of things you hate about being overweight and the pain it's causing you. Now get in touch with those painful feelings and memories and use them as motivation to change. When you read over this list of painful reasons, say to yourself all these may be causing me pain right now but I can change back to pleasure. That pleasure is not going to come not from those bad habits, but from getting on the exercise bike or pushing that plate away before you're full.

Personally I prefer positive motivation but if negative motivation works for you, use it. Put a list of those negative things close to hand. This way, you'll be reminded of the pain that this weight gain is causing you. This way whenever you're feeling less motivated than you should be, a quick glance we remind you and motivate you to take action.

Here's what "M.O.M.E.N.T.U.M" means to me...

M - Momentum - The only way to keep momentum and motivation going is to have constantly greater goals, start small and build on your successes!

O - Organize - Organize your life (both time and space) so you never need excuses for not exercising.

T - Take Any Small Step - Every journey starts with a single step and every small step towards your goals feeds your motivation.

I - Identify - Identify the behaviors that you need to change. The person you are is because of the behaviors you currently have, so what behavior do you need to change to become that new person?

V - Visualize - Visualize your goal frequently for 5-10 minutes. Picture success in your mind and the life that's coming to you. Martin Luther King Jr had a dream, what's yours?

A - Active Mind - You can have an active body without an active mind. Take care of your mind with a proper diet and sleep and you will have the physical stamina to maintain the momentum.

T - Thoughts - To stay motivated you need to stay positive in your thoughts. Successful dieters turn the negative events that are sure to occur into learning experiences, then they adjust accordingly and move on.

I - Inspiration - Find inspiration, on a daily basis. Read inspiring stories of others who were on the path as you and succeeded, they will help you to gain confidence that you too can also do it.

O - Online/Offline Help - Find a group of people online/offline that you inspire and motivate you to succeed

N - Never Skip 2 Days In A Row - There will be times you miss the odd workout day here and there, but never skip more than 2, or you may lose the head of steam you've built up.

Now on to that other dieting gremlin that ruins diets for most people, emotional eating...

HOW TO GET CONTROL OF EMOTIONAL EATING

"Know your enemy and know yourself and you can fight a hundred battles without disaster" - Sun Tzu

You're probably wondering why I've started this chapter with this quote, but I think it appropriate for what we're about to talk about. There are a lot of people who train hard, watch what they eat and would love to have a greater figure, but are held back by emotional eating. But, if you know your enemy (emotional eating) better, it's easier to put up a better fight when those triggers kick in. If you're tired of emotional eating, then here's what you need to do in order win this war. In most cases stress, loneliness, sadness, or lack of self-confidence is the emotions to blame for emotional eating.

Stress & Emotional Eating

If you eat due to stress, why not take up yoga or meditation to calm yourself. If you eat out of loneliness, sign up for a course or a class of some sort to be around people and make new friends. When you begin taking action to reduce the control your emotions have on you, your cravings will also diminish. It will take time and practice, but if you do this regularly, you will have a lot more control over what you eat and how much you eat.

Social Situations & Emotional Eating Triggers

Social situations can also be a trigger for emotional eating; you may find that you eat when you're not hungry because you're encouraged by others to do so. You may see an advertisement for a particular food that reminds you of a happy memory (associated with that food), which then causes you to crave it and consume it. Or you may pass your favorite restaurant or bakery and sit down for a meal even when you're not hungry. Emotional eating can also stem from food's association with certain activities like going to the movies, attending a sporting event, or simply just watching television.

Is Your Hunger Real or Caused By Emotion?

But how can you tell when you are truly hungry or perhaps just experiencing a non-hunger food craving? When a craving for a certain high-calorie food strikes, stop and think. Your brain may say, "I need a candy bar now" but instead think, is there a healthier real food option that would stop this hunger. If this sound good then you're probably hungry, but if all you want is the high-calorie snack and nothing else, you know who's to blame.

Is Your Emotional Craving Caused By Something Physical?

While you might think all emotional eating stems from mental causes there also can be a physical reason. For example if someone is feeling bad for whatever reason, the body reacts by trying to produce more serotonin (the brain's natural feel good hormone) to balance things out. But, because carbohydrates also can increase the level of serotonin, your body craves those "potato chips, ice cream and chocolate" as a short cut to restoring your emotional equilibrium.

8 Ways to Overcome Emotional Overeating

With emotional eating triggers, the important thing to remember is to try to consciously notice the food triggers and the feelings they create. When you start to notice them at a conscious level, it stops them from sneaking into your subconscious mind unnoticed, and they lose their power to take control of you and your eating.

Here are 8 other ways to get to grips with emotional overeating...

1 - Write Down Your Craving - The next time you get a craving for a particular food write it down, include the time of day and what you were doing at the time of the craving.

This helps for these 3 reasons,

   * You can spot which food is causing the problem and avoid having it in your home or workplace.

   * You may notice a pattern between what you're doing at that moment and the craving...this way you can either avoid doing the particular thing or do something else till the craving passes.

* And it can help take the urge of the craving away!

2 - Limited Your Intake - If your craving is soooo bad and you can't avoid it, then limit your intake to only 2 bites and throw the rest away. This way you get your fix, without the extra calories you don't really need.

3 - Remember Food Won't Make the World A Better Place - Is there a link between your emotional over eating and a crisis at home, money worries, kids playing up? While your craving may make the world a better place for a few moments, unfortunately it can't turn your life around. It's better to go for a healthier option to coping with stress, this way you don't have the added guilt for overindulging yourself later on.

4 - How Is Food Limiting Your Life - A good way to take the power away from a craving/emotional over eating is to write a list of things you can't do, because of that extra weight.

* Is your weight preventing you getting out and about?

* Does it limit what activities you can do - like not being able to play with your kids?

* Is it causing other health problems?

* Is it affecting your social life, meeting members of the opposite sex, etc?

Now keep that list at hand and refer to it when your cravings starts. Would eating that piece of chocolate cake really mean more to you than overcoming these limitations?

5 - Stop Eating Alone - To overcome a pattern of overeating, make a promise to stop eating alone. This way you can share your treat and eat less, and also become more conscious of your eating habits.

6 - Record Your Successes - Buy yourself a diary and at the end of the day record those successes/small achievements you've had that day. It mightn't seem much but it's a great way of looking back on your days/weeks/months and seeing how your eating habits have improved. It helps to remind you that you're closer to becoming that healthy slimmer person you want to be.

7 - Don't Feel Guilty About Wasting Food - If you're one of those people who feels guilty about throwing food in the garbage can, you need to stop thinking like this. It's not doing your health and waistline any good. Clearing all those last scraps of food off everyone's plate, is just transferring that waste from the bin to your hips. Remember your bins not going to have to work out to burn the excess weight off, you will!

8 - Set Small Goals - Rome wasn't built in a day and you can't expect to become a brand new person overnight. Pick some smaller goals and aim to achieve those first, then when you can easily do these, move on to the bigger ones.

Reasons for Emotional Overeating

Some people say that solving emotional overeating is as easy as just telling people to stop being lazy, exercise, and stop over eating. But for many, food means so many more things other than fuel for their. The mind can be a powerful thing and the craving for food can become so intense that stopping it is like trying to stop a monster, with only food being the way which you can find solace and emotional peace.

But, is the mind the only cause of overeating or are other reasons....

   * Studies have shown that women who go undiagnosed as ADD (but do in fact have it) are much more likely to develop an Eating Disorder. Some of the neurological symptoms of ADD/ADHD can be: holding onto negative thoughts and/or anger, as well as impulsivity both verbally (interrupting others) and in actions (acting before thinking).

* Stress – In an America poll, more than 80 percent of Americans say money and the economy are two significant stressors in their lives. With nearly half admitting that they use overeating to cope.

   * Many children - like adults - eat for comfort, often because of self-dislike, difficulties with school work or friendlessness. This loneliness is then made worse when a child is shunned and bullied simply for being fat.

   * Associated with rare conditions such as Prader-Willi Syndrome (PWS), hyperphagia can cause a person to overeat excessively -- even sneaking or stealing food in an attempt to satisfy their unstoppable hunger. About

4,500 Americans are diagnosed with PWS, but experts believe that undiagnosed cases would raise the total to nearly 30,000.

Tips for Overcoming Emotional Overeating

If you can see a pattern in your moods, your eating and dieting cycles, you can pinpoint the triggers of your overeating. Just as alcoholics and other drug abusers are advised to avoid situations where the object of their addiction is easily accessible, emotional eaters need to be aware of how the behavior of others can influence their tendency to overindulge.

Thanksgiving dinners (the stress of a large family gathering coupled with an abundance of enticing entrees) and wedding receptions (lots of happy people eating lots of delicious cake) are all situations in which the spirit of the crowd can sweep us away from our healthy eating goals.

If you feel emotional tendencies increasing, there are some things you can do to keep your mind off the topic of food or when you're upset...

* Blow off steam by going for a run or take the dog out for a walk.

* Call a friend, read a book or go for a walk in the mall.

* Eat lots of water laden food, juicy fruit and or vegetables can be very filling on the stomach without the high calorie levels.

* Treat yourself to a new body lotion or a new book or magazine, something that can cheer you up/keep you occupied.

Try to figure out what kinds of situations you encounter regularly that cause you to overeat?

By identifying your triggers, habits, and vulnerabilities you're on the first step towards breaking the cycle. Then try to build good habits, establish a healthy relationship with food and give your body the care it deserves. For people suffering from emotional overeating they have to learn how to eat 'intuitively.' This means letting your body tell you when you're hungry, instead of listening to your mind. But if you do snack when you're feeling emotional, don't let that mistake pull your mood down even further. Remember to look at it for what it is, try to find the triggers or the reason behind the problem and you're well on your way to getting control of your eating.

While emotional eating could be telling you what to eat, let's take a look at how your food could be making your eating decisions for you...

How TO CONQUER FOOD AND SUGAR CRAVINGS

There are times when we all reach for some type of comfort food and after a few mouthfuls the world seems like a better place. But now scientists believe that the secret behind comfort foods is all in the mind, as foods that are high in sugar and fat can alter the chemicals in the brain and help us to relax. Foods high in carbohydrates like pasta raise levels of serotonin in the brain and so make us feel better. It seems that high levels of stress in early life can change how nerves form in the brain and foods high in sugar or fat help to balance these changes and make us feel better.

In research done on rats they found that those who underwent stress in the beginning of their lives had higher stress levels than normal. But when these rats were fed fattening foods their levels of stress and anxious behavior dropped. So, if you feel guilty for reaching for that candy bar don't put it down to poor will power, you now know there are other things at play here.

7 Things You Should Know About Food Cravings.

Food cravings can affect even the most determined dieter and can mean different things to different people. For example you can have the "harmless" cravings for things like chocolate, starchy foods like French fries, to the harmful non-food substances like clay, laundry starch or other items.

So how what causes them and how can you conquer food cravings? Here's seven things to keep in mind...

1 – Food cravings can be a sign of low blood sugar and/or a diet too low in calories. Remember don't starve yourself as this is most likely to lead to you experience cravings, and to give in to temptation.

2 – Sometimes giving in to a craving is a better solution than avoiding it. For example women who tried to stop thinking about chocolate, ate 50% more than those who were encouraged to talk about their cravings. The women who had tried to suppress their cravings, ate on average eight chocolates, while those who had talked freely about it ate only five.

3 – Emotions can have an effect on food cravings – If you feel low try to find a healthier way to improve your state. Try some of the examples given previously, as a low mood or feeling tired means low serotonin which can lead to a craving for sugar and/or carbohydrates.

4 – Food cravings and so called comfort food cravings are often really just stress signals misinterpreted. For example if foods with pleasurable tastes and textures were used as a reward or to provide solace during childhood, then the psychological component for craving such foods grows even stronger.

5 – There's is a difference between food craving and food addictions, food addiction is a serious problem and should be treated by a physician and/or dietician as soon as it's identified.

6 – Drink plenty of water as dehydration can sometimes be mistaken for hunger and can increase cravings, especially for sweet foods.

7 – If you crave ice cream, have a scoop instead of eating too much of something "healthy." It may sound like you're cheating on your diet, but giving in a little bit is a lot better than going without over a long period and then pigging out! This won't do your diet or confidence any good.

In many ways, treatment of food addictions is similar to drug and alcohol addiction. The first step to recovery is recognizing and accepting the problem, and identifying which foods cause symptoms and cravings. However, unlike drug and alcohol addiction, food addicts can't quit cold turkey. Instead of taking drastic measures, make the following changes gradually, one small step at a time.

1 – Sweet foods are a problem area for food addicts. As you crave foods that are laden with sugar, your taste buds get used to the flavor and you start craving sweeter and sweeter foods. To cut back on this problem they to avoid buying foods that aren't supposed to be sweet, like pasta sauce, bread and crackers. Believe it or not, just these products alone contain added sweeteners like fructose, dextrose, and corn syrup.

2 – Avoid having foods you crave in your house, car or somewhere you can get to them in a hurry. It may sound like a simple thing to do, but not

having those foods around keeps temptation at bay. It also gives you the opportunity to solve your problem other than relying on food.

3 – Food addiction is a fake hunger and to get over this problem, you need to become aware of what you are eating. The best way to do this is to maintain a food journal. In your food journal list when and what you eat during the day, and how it makes you feel. Over time you'll notice trends, foods and situations that are to blame for your problem.

4 – Remember that food addiction is a short circuit to feeling better. But it is also a short circuit in another sense, the more you use this mechanism, the more you bypass ways of managing your feelings. Relying on food won't make those problems go away and they will return another day, if you don't come to terms with them. The more you avoid taking action, the more you need the cure, which makes you eat more of what you shouldn't.

5 – People with food addiction often overeat because the signals that traditionally tell the body to stop eating don't happen. To solve this problem retrain your brain to feel full on less food, by using smaller plates and bowls which force you to dish out smaller portions.

6 – The internet can also be a very helpful way of finding online support groups and clubs to help food addicts or compulsive eaters. Two very useful resource groups and websites to help food addicts are "Overeaters Anonymous" and "Food Addicts In Recovery Anonymous". Both programs are based on the twelve steps and twelve traditions of alcoholics anonymous.

Now that we've talked about food cravings, let's take a look at the white stuff you could be addicted to...

SUGAR ADDICTION – ARE YOU ADDICTED TO THE WHITE STUFF?

Our natural instinct is to appreciate sweet tastes, which begins from birth with the taste of sweet breast milk. But times have changed and the majority of modern diets involve sugar in some form or other. Sugar is very difficult to avoid nowadays as its included in most prepared and prepackaged foods we all eat. From the obvious soft drinks and alcohol, to salad dressings and condiments, sugar is involved in most foods either for taste or as a preservative. Addiction to sugar is not the result of a mental disorder, character flaw or weak will. The roots of sugar addiction, as well as any other addiction, lie in neurotransmitters in the reward pathway of the brain.

Sugar addiction develops in several different ways. Partly it is due to the fact that sugar effects the area in the brain called the reward pathway in the same manner as drugs and alcohol, it over stimulates the neurotransmitters until they no longer function properly. This tolerance then develops and the mind becomes dependent more and more on sugar to function. Additionally, because sugar is void of any nutritional value, the body never gets the chromium and other essential nutrients it needs and therefore it keeps craving more.

However addiction to sugar can also be due to fact that you're allergic or sensitive to it. When you're allergic or sensitive to a food you often develop an addiction to it. An addiction to anything including sugar is something that we do in order to avoid a negative feeling or symptom.

People use sugar as a comfort food and a form of self-medication, but because addictions tend to deteriorate our bodies, we often feel better with the addictive substance, but the end result is usually that we feel worse as can't perform as best as we should. For example, sugar temporarily increases energy and elevates happiness and a feeling of well-being. But after a period of blood sugar spikes, there is a drop in blood sugar or a sugar crash which leaves the person lethargic and needing another pick me up.

If you feel that you may suffer from a sugar addiction make the decision to try to stop eating it completely for at least 4 days. Although the longer the better you will feel if you stick to it. While I usually recommend making small changes gradually to your diet, sugar has the unique ability to inspire cravings which are refueled every time you give into them. The only way to break the cycle is to stop feeding the fire. Once your sugar tolerance has normalized you can reintroduce it in small amounts, so long as you are sure you are eating for pleasure and not from habit. If you hope to get through it, you must have a strategy for diverting yourself from temptation.

Start by removing all sweets (especially your weakness) from the house. If you do not want to throw things out, try giving them away at work or even sealing them up and putting them somewhere you can't get to them. Making it impossible to cheat will greatly increase your probability of success.

Then try to introduce fruit or vegetables that have a sweet flavor that can satisfy your sweet tooth but don't have hidden sugars. Other ways to overcome a sugar addiction are to keep a food journal, living by strict dietary menus and taking cooking classes to learn how to make low-sugar or sugar-free meals. If you feel that you do have a big problem with sugar the best advice I would give is to get in touch with your doctor or health practioner who can guide you on the best practices that will work for you.

If you do feel you have a problem with sugar here are....

10 Sugar Craving Tips

1 – Sugar cravings can be a sign of hormonal imbalances due to a nutritional deficiency in the body. A poor diet or hormonal imbalance can cause you to feel tired or a little down and you reach for sugar as a "pick me up."

2 – Replace the sweets you are consuming with healthy alternatives, such as fruit. They taste sweet, will supplement your sugar cravings but will not have the same negative effects on your body as sugar, which is empty of nutrients and vitamins.

3 – Find ways to fulfill your cravings for sweets without giving up sweets entirely. Instead of eating an entire candy bar, replace it with a "fun" size candy bar (but make sure you stick to one only).

4 – Eating too quickly can also cause your blood sugar levels to rise quickly. This means that your blood sugar levels will decrease sooner making you feel hungry again. By eating your meals slowly, helps you avoid these spikes in blood sugar levels, and possible sugar cravings.

5 – Switch to wholegrain foods such as wholegrain bread, pasta and rice. As the body processes the over refined and over processed white flour as sugar, it can affect you the same way sugar does.

6 – Identify your triggers for sugar cravings and then try to avoid them. Common triggers for sugar cravings are boredom, lack of energy and stress. Try to find alternative ways of dealing with these triggers and you'll be well on the path to beating your sugar cravings.

7 – Scientists believe that we instinctively reach for food that increases the "happiness hormone" (serotonin) and one of the fastest ways is with sugar. Sugar is the body's quickest source of energy and can change our mood in seconds. If you're feeling down find a healthier way to raise serotonin levels, with some exercise like a short walk.

8 – Some people report that having some protein instead of sugar when the cravings hit helps to quieten down their cravings.

9 – One of the most common causes of sugar cravings is irregular eating. If you skip meals or eat on an unpredictable schedule, this can result in catapulting your body into a state of starvation. As a result, your body sends out messages that it needs energy in a hurry and sends out sugar cravings. The easy solution to this is to make sure that you are eating more frequent, smaller meals each day.

10 - You might think you've taken as much sugar out of your diet already but sugar comes in various guises that you might not know. Here are other names for sugar on food labels - corn syrup, demerara sugar, dextrose, free flowing brown sugars, fructose, galactose, glucose, high fructose corn syrup, invert sugar, lactose, malt, molasses, maple syrup, sucrose, and maltose.

BUT while you may think sugar causes food cravings, don't rule out the problems salt can cause you...

Is Salt To Blame For Your Food Cravings?

Do you feel compelled to add an extra pinch of salt to your foods even before you taste them; chances are you've got an addiction to salt. But rather than adding salt to food for the added spice it gives to your food, you're probably adding it to because it puts you in a better mood.

According to researchers in the University of Iowa people who go without salt for long periods can become depressed. They found that adding salt to their diet, puts people in a better mood and creates cravings comparable to a drug addiction. Although some salt in needed in the body to help fluids pass through the body, too much can cause health problems like high blood pressure and heart disease.

Professor Kim Johnson who did tests on rats, found that when salt levels were lowered they lost the pleasure in drinking sugary drinks. They also noticed a similar change in brain activity when the rats were denied drugs. "This suggests that salt need and cravings, may be linked to the same brain pathways as those related to drug addiction and abuse," Prof Johnson added.

While some people out there may say that obesity is a matter of poor will power, it seems that manufacturers of food are designing food to become more addictive and salt seems to be a great way of doing this. While we all know the dangers of eating too much sugary foods, salt hasn't gotten as much press until lately, with ads on British TV highlighting the fact of high salt content in foods.

As with sugar, salt is routinely added to our foods and we don't even notice it. Salt is now added to almost all types of food and camouflaged with high levels of sugar to sweeten the taste. This is probably why a portion of salty French fries tastes so good when it's washed down with your favorite soda drink. The salt gives us an initial hit and heightens the feelings of the sugary taste of the soda.

If you think about it we've allowed our food to dictate to us what we should eat rather than the other way around. So the next time you get a craving for something sweet think back, was that last food that I ate high in salt content? Chances are it was, and know you know where that cravings coming from!

We've looked at how fat can control how, and what you eat, but did you know it can also burn fat...?

HOW TO USE FOOD TO BURN FAT

"Burning fat", what image does that create in your mind, hours spent slumped over a treadmill or exercise bike in the hope of burning some calories? Well forget all that, because you're about to discover how to use the food we eat every day to burn that ugly belly fat.

Fat burning foods get their title due to the way they burn fat in the body, and or improve your metabolism (the rate as which your body burns calories). The best bit is they do all of this without you even breaking out in a sweat.

Let's take a look at breakfast for an example. To most people breakfast is easily overlooked as the best time to boost their metabolism and fat burning. In numerous studies done all over the world it's been found again and again that people who eat breakfast, have better eating habits, weigh less and eat less calories in their day.

If you consider the image of your metabolism as a huge furnace that burns 24 hours a day, 7 days a week, you'll see that to keep that fire roaring at all times, is in your interest. Our bodies metabolism works in cycles, at night it slows down (because our body goes into repair mode), and during the day it speeds up (to give us energy to move around and also to help digest the food we've eaten that day).

But and this is a big but, if you don't give your body breakfast first thing in the morning, your metabolism doesn't get a chance to pick up, and it remains in slow motion for the rest of the day. The very fact of eating, breaking down and digesting food, increases our metabolism and calories burnt for the rest of the day. Then add to that the fact, that your body has more energy to work with and you can see that skipping breakfast, rather making you slimmer is in fact making you fatter.

If it's been a while since you've been in the habit of eating breakfast, you will need to change your morning routine. If sitting down to a meal straight after getting up is difficult, start your morning with a glass of water. This helps to boost metabolism (a slow metabolism is linked to a dehydrated body) and gives your stomach a wakeup call that food isn't too far away.

TIP – Just as a side note if you can, try to drink a glass of cold water (even iced) first thing. Our bodies don't like working with cold foods and need to increase that food up to the body temperature before it can use it. This heating up (just like a kettle heating up water), uses more calories than just drinking plain old tap water at room temperature.

After you've drank your glass of water, go about your normal routine but leave yourself an extra 10 -15 minutes to eat some breakfast before going out the door. Here are some simple and quick breakfast food ideas.

-   A piece of fruit or yogurt
-   A meal replacement drink (quick easy to prepare)
-   Breakfast or cereal bar. (If you do use this option, read the ingredient label for sugar and fat levels. Most modern breakfast and protein bars and biscuits are loaded with sugar.)

When choosing a breakfast cereal for breakfast, pay attention to food labels. Like breakfast bars, most contain sugars and other ingredients that your body doesn't need. When checking out food labels, pay attention to the quantity of fiber (which should be five grams or more per serving), less than eight grams of sugar per serving and sugar shouldn't be in the first three ingredients on the list.

Here are 3 popular fat burning foods...

1 - Caffeine - Caffeine has been used for years by runners and endurance people to enhance fatty acid metabolism. It's particularly effective in those who are not habitual users. When it is in your blood stream, caffeine tends to keep fatty enzyme in your blood for longer, which causes your metabolism to burn them instead of storing them. Caffeine also has the unique ability to enhance the effects of other fat burning compounds like green tea and citrus aurantium. When combined in a multi-ingredient diet formula, caffeine can play a critical role in improving the effectiveness of a diet and exercise program.

In a study done on caffeine and fat burning, one group taking green tea or tyrosine experienced almost no increase in metabolic rate. While those who were in another group taking only 50 mgs of caffeine experienced anywhere from a three to 16 percent increase in thermogenesis (the rate one burns calories).

2 - Apple Cider Vinegar - If you can get over the taste of apple cider vinegar, you will find it one of the most important natural remedies in healing the body. Apple cider vinegar has been used as a weight loss remedy for centuries, and although the mechanics are not always clear on how it works, it really does seem to work. But whatever the reason, the fact remains that it has stood the test of time as a fat-busting supplement, and has helped countless people to achieve their ideal weight. As far back as 3,000 BC, Egyptians were using it for health benefits including weight loss and Hippocrates, the father of modern medicine, was said to have used cider vinegar for its healing qualities.

Apple cider vinegar seems to work because it speeds up the metabolism especially when taken regularly before meals, and if used in conjunction with a sensible diet and exercise program, it can be a powerful aid in keeping your weight under control. It's probably also the best (and cheapest) detoxifier for the body. It helps to detoxify the liver and break down fat and helps with digesting rich, fatty and greasy foods, and also for proper metabolizing of proteins, fats and minerals.

Is Apple Cider Vinegar Safe and How Do You Use It?

You may safely add apple cider vinegar to food and/or drinking water, starting with small amounts and building up to ½ to 1 teaspoon per 15 pounds of body weight or about 1 tsp. apple cider vinegar (health food store variety best) to 8oz. water before every meal. If you want to lose weight using apple cider vinegar, I'd recommend that you drink 2-3 glasses of extra water daily to help your body flush this fat out and speed up the weight loss process. Apple cider vinegar is also said to contain an abundance of complex carbohydrates and dietary fiber. Adding more fiber to your diet (such as the pectin in apple cider vinegar), helps to assist our body by having regular bowel movements and proper elimination.

How Does Apple Cider Vinegar Help With Weight Loss?

Apple cider vinegar improves digestion which in turn reduces the amount of time that fats remain in the digestive tract. The less time fats are present in the digestive tract, the less fats will be absorbed and the greater the weight loss. It has been suggested that the apple cider vinegar works because it makes the body burn calories better, that it reduces the appetite, or simply that it gets the entire metabolism working at top efficiency. It also promotes digestion, assimilation and elimination and it neutralizes any toxic substance taken into the body.

Apple cider vinegar has been used for centuries in aiding the liver to detoxify the body and to help with digesting rich, fatty and greasy foods, and for proper metabolizing of proteins, fats and minerals. Some people claim that the regular consumption of an apple cider vinegar tonic makes body fat disappear because the vinegar helps curb appetite and causes fat to be burned instead of stored.

The combination of the acidic vinegar and fruit pectin is supposedly the reason behind this solution's "fat burning effects". It's also rich in acetic, malic and tartaric acids, natural compounds that help the liver break down cortisol, insulin and other fat storing hormones.

Although the jury may be out on the weight loss benefits of cider vinegar, some even go as far as to call it a fad diet, I disagree. For the thousands of people who take it, not only with losing weight but also for their symptoms of arthritis, joint pain, gout, diverticulitis and other troublesome complaints. It's a simple and cheap health ingredient to add to your shopping list. As the old saying goes "An apple a day can keep the doctor away" so imagine what a bottle of cider of vinegar might do for you?

3 - Green Tea - Green tea has been used by the Chinese and Japanese for centuries. It is described as a miracle drink that is able to cure or even prevent certain kinds of illnesses. Even today, you can find it being offered by traditional Chinese herbal pharmacists as a form of medicine. It has been known to prevent diabetes, cancer, as well as a cure for bad breath. However, did you know that this tea can also help in weight loss?

Green tea contains minerals and vitamins that help in stabilizing your metabolism rate, help in extracting energy from food faster and also to burns more fats faster. By increasing the metabolism rate and increasing the amount of energy from food, green tea helps to make you feel more active and energetic. Another key benefit of green tea is that it is an appetite suppressant which helps in weight loss. This can be used by drinking green tea dinner, which should help to suppress your appetite and avoid overeating during dinner. This is why green tea is also known as a slimming tea by the Chinese. It's no surprise that the Japanese and the Chinese don't have a lot of overweight people.

10 Fat Burning Foods That You Can Find In Your Kitchen

1 – Lime, lemons, oranges – Contain high levels of Vitamin C and flavones which help to burn fat, and the added fiber from the fruit offers a huge benefit as it helps to fill you up and reduce your calorie intake.

2 – Avocados – This wonder fruit helps fat burning due to its high concentrations of monounsaturated fat specifically oleic acid, which is also found in macadamia nut oil. Not only does this type of fat turn on your fat burners it also lowers LDL cholesterol and triglycerides.

3 – Eggs – Eggs have received a bad rap in the past due to the high cholesterol content. However recent studies show that dietary cholesterol has little effect on blood cholesterol. Eggs are high in protein and vitamin B12 both of which help to burn fat. They're also the most basic of proteins which make you fuller with fewer calories.

4 – Berries – Raspberries, strawberries, blueberries and blackberries are a good quality source of vitamins, minerals, antioxidants and even fiber, which can help to control blood sugar and cravings.

5 – Water – Drink ice cold water. German researchers have found dieters can increase their metabolic rate by as much as 30% by drinking 17 ounces of cold water.

6 – Caffeine – Caffeine helps to jump-starts lipolysis, the breakdown of fat. One to two cups a day is ideal, but don't get carried away. Having too much can increase your blood pressure, and may make you feel nervous and jittery.

7 – Grapefruit – Scientists discovered that eating half a grapefruit three times a day before each meal helped people lose an additional 3.6 pounds over twelve weeks, without changing their diet in any other way.

8 – Milk – Milk is a rich source of complex carbohydrates, which can boost your metabolism by helping to keep insulin levels low after meals (low insulin levels are desirable as high insulin levels are the signal to your body to hang onto fat). In an article published by the Obesity Research clinic found that females that consumed low fat dairy foods, like low fat milk at least 3 - 4 times daily, burned 70 percent more body fat compared to low dairy eaters.

9 – Garlic – Garlic, garlic oil, or anything with garlic, has an antibiotic property to it and can be used to cure many ailments. Another little known benefit of garlic is that it has the power to reduce fat levels in your cells.

10 – Lean Meats – The protein in lean meats can help in increasing your metabolic rate after ingestion, this is due to the extra work your body has to do digest them compared to carbohydrates or fats. Some examples of lean meats are boneless, skinless chicken, turkey, lean beef, salmon, tuna, and other fish that is broiled or baked.

While this chapter is based on the topic of fat burning foods, I thought I'd also include a page or two on the topic of other foods that are also important in weight loss, and that's...

Negative Calorie Foods

Negative calorie foods are foods that require more calories for the body to digest them, than the calories they give back in return. For example, if you consider water to be a food, then cold water is certainly a negative calorie food. It gives no calories, but the body has to expend energy to bring it up to body temperature. So every time a glass of cold water is drank, some of the bodies calories are used up in the process.

NOTE - Negative calorie foods are very attractive to anorexics and other people who suffer from eating disorders, and for that reason I would like to give a warning here first. A negative calorie diet would obviously result in starvation in the long term and nutritional deficiencies can occur surprisingly quickly. The calories burnt usually come from muscle mass, and the result is debility and wasting.

A more healthy way to use a negative calorie diet is as a form of fasting or detox. Something for example, that can be done for one to three days right after the Christmas season or another time when you have been eating an over-rich diet. Provided you are otherwise healthy it can be a great way to clean out the system. However it is still best to take medical advice before attempting this.

If you decide to use a negative calorie detox, keep the following points in mind:

1. It is never a good idea to eat huge quantities of one type of food, especially fruits. A lot of foods can contain elements that can be damaging if consumed to excess. For example, the acid in grapefruit and pineapple can damage your stomach lining. Other foods may put an excessive burden on the liver or may cause diarrhea. So try to use a variety of different foods in small quantities.

2. Do not spend all day eating negative calorie foods as you'll possibly end up feeling bloated and/or sick. Plan four or five salad meals each day, and let your digestion rest at other times.

3. You will feel more satisfied if you eat slowly and chew your food thoroughly. You will also use more calories that way. If the foods are eaten raw, that will be more effective and won't lose nutrients than cooking them. Foods like carrots and beets can also be more satisfying if you eat them grated.

4. Schedule time when you do not have any important commitments. As with fasting or any kind of detox, you may suffer some uncomfortable symptoms including headaches, tiredness, depression and irritability. If these become severe, stop the diet, return to your normal diet and if needed see your doctor.

5. When you end the detox, plan a gradual return to normal eating.

If all the above points are checked and passed, let's move on to the list of foods...

Apples

Asparagus

Beets

Blueberries

Broccoli

Cantaloupes

Carrot

Cauliflower

Celery stalk

Celery root

Cranberries

Cucumbers

Eggplant

Endives

Garden cress

Garlic

Grapefruit

Green beans

Green cabbage

Lamb's lettuce

Lemons

Lettuce

Onions

Papayas

Pineapples

Prunes

Radishes

Raspberries

Spinach

Strawberries

Tangerines

Tomatoes

Turnips

Zucchini.

Now that we've looked at food cravings, emotional eating and negative calories, what happens if suddenly you stop losing weight...?

HOW TO OVERCOME WEIGHT LOSS PLATEAUS

Where once you were very happy with the results you were getting, suddenly after a month or two, you may notice that your weight loss is getting slower and slower, until it finally grinds to a halt. You my dieting friend, have probably just hit that hidden weight loss wall, the weight loss plateau. So what is a weight loss plateau and how do you get over or around it?

A weight loss plateau is a normal part of losing weight and has a good scientific explanation. A plateau occurs when you are in energy balance, stalling out means leptin levels have dropped to the point where fat loss is extremely difficult if not impossible. This usually happens when you drop calories more and more over a period of time.

Another way to look at weight loss plateaus is that they are actually your body settling in at a new body weight set point. The set point theory is basically the idea that your body likes to be at a certain body weight and it will work to keep you there. Weight loss plateaus are frustrating but don't let them discourage you or stop you from reaching your goal.

Here are 7 reasons why you may be suffering from a weight loss plateau…

1 – Your body may have got used to your exercise routine and doesn't burn as many calories as it used to. So in order to deal with such a weight loss plateau, you need to change what you're doing either by exercising longer or doing a different form of fat burning activity.

2 – Be especially careful about "low-fat" foods where flavour is enhanced by sugar and other carbohydrates this can add hidden calories to your daily intake.

3 – If you aren't getting enough sleep, or not eating enough food (or the right combination of complex carbs, healthy fats and protein, this can stall your progress.

4 – As your weight goes down, you not only lose fat but also a small amount of muscle. Since muscle is critical to keeping your metabolism

revved, losing it can reduce your metabolic rate and hinder your weight loss.

5 – If you're on a low calorie diet this could be the reason for your plateau. Try alternating higher-calorie days with lower-calorie days. By mixing up your daily intake— say you eat 1800 calories on Monday, and then 2100 calories on Tuesday—you'll keep your body guessing and avoid that plateau.

6 – Look for places that calories tend to hide such as dressings, sauces, and condiments. If cutting out any more food isn't an option, you'll need to up your workout activity. Many studies show that small, frequent meals are more satisfying and produce better weight-loss results than the same number of calories consumed in three large meals. Take advantage of healthy snacking and crunch on fresh slices of raw vegetables like celery, peppers and cucumber when you're hungry.

7 – Dining out typically means much higher fat content (and therefore calorie content), as well as very large portion sizes. Try to limit how often you dine out or order takeout food. Unless you are good at maths, it can be hard to figure out how many grams of energy (kilojoules), fat or sugar can be in each meal.

Exercise should first on your list to get over a weight loss plateau, because it increases the metabolic rate and burns calories. Some researchers believe that the metabolic increase persists for several hours beyond the exercise period. Cutting back even further on calories will send the body the wrong message. Remember: When you rob the cells of energy, the body immediately goes into conservation mode and stores energy.

Weight loss plateaus are probably among the most frustrating obstacles for dieters, you feel like you're doing everything right and trying your hardest and the scale just won't budge. But they can also help you in many different ways by suggesting the proper dieting techniques or the proper balanced blend of foods that you should be eating. And they can also help to let you know what harm you may be doing to your body.

But while you might be suffering from a weight loss plateau did you know that…

Your Bathroom Scales Could Be Telling Lies?

It can be a useful tool or your worst enemy. Many women have a love-hate relationship with their bathroom scale, dreading to step onto its flat, shiny surface to see what number it will spit back at them.

But even though it may give you a figure in black and white, sometimes it's not always telling the truth!

Here are 4 reasons why your bathroom scales are telling fibs...

1 - On digital bathroom scales, low batteries and faulty AC adapters can be the number 1 cause of scale malfunction and inaccuracy. A scale will perform slowly, or read inaccurately when it has low batteries. A faulty AC adapter can cause your scale to act unstable with numbers "jumping" all over the place. If you're not sure replace your batteries with good quality ones and check if you find a difference in results.

2 - Not all bathroom scales are created equal. If you have an old spring type "analog" bathroom scales throw it out. It may have been right on the mark when you bought it but over time it loses its accuracy. Go for digital scales instead as they're more accurate and have other great functions like measuring body fat as well.

3 - If you've been drinking a lot of water over a period of time, your body tends not to hold onto much as it knows it's in plentiful supply. But cut back on your water intake and you may find your weight creeping up due to water retention, sometimes even by a few pounds.

To undo this, just return to your former water drinking routine and you'll find those pounds just drop away again. Also watch your salt intake, it's nearly impossible to find any type of processed food that doesn't contain salt, even sweet foods have in abundance. This salt then makes your body prone to water retention and you look heavier on the scale the next morning.

4 - Glycogen levels can also affect your weight. Glycogen is a fuel made up of carbohydrates, which the body stores in reserve in the liver and muscles. When reserves are full it can weigh up to 3-4 pounds including water. But if you don't eat as much carbohydrates as usual, your body

works from these stores thus making you lighter. It's possible to suddenly go down a few pounds very quickly without even changing your daily activity or calorie intake.

But the opposite is also true; start to eat more carbohydrates (your body fills these stores again) and suddenly you're a few pounds heavier for no apparent reason.

Finally, never, ever, try out bathroom scales other than your own. You may be tempted to try out a friends when visiting the loo but don't. You'll only get a different reading, upset yourself and think your scales are wrong or maybe right, if yours say you're lighter. :)

Just stick to using your own bathroom scales this way you've got a more accurate idea of how you're progressing. But if you have the cash to spare, splash out on a good quality scales that give a body fat reading as well as record your weight. You'll be able to see if you're really on the right path and losing fat rather than losing muscle!

Just stick to using your own bathroom scales this way you've got a more accurate idea of how you're progressing. But if you have the cash to spare, splash out on a good quality scales that give a body fat reading as well as record your weight. You'll be able to see if you're really on the right path and losing fat rather than losing muscle!

34 EASY WAYS TO REDUCE CALORIES

1- Reduce all your serving plates by 20%. Over time your brain and stomach will get used to the difference.
2- While is good for you, unfortunately the fat isn't. An easy way to reduce cheese calories is to zap your cheese in a microwave oven, and then pour off the grease.
3- Try drinking a glass or orange juice half or one hour before meal times. The fructose in the fruit can help to supress your appetite.
4- Try to avoid trans fatty acids when cooking. Corn oil, olive or canola is a much healthier option when preparing meals.
5- Use fruit purees in place of margarine or butter. They can be easily prepared in a food processor and help to lower fat and calories.
6- Try sticking to only 4 egg yolks per week to cut down on add fat.
7- Change your milk drinking habits from full fat to half fat or skimmed. It may take a while for your taste buds to get used to it but it's another easy to reduce calories.
8- Substitute all Hollandaise, Alfredo and cream based sauces for tomato based ones. They're lower in calories. You can also season your food with lemon or low calorie soy sauce for flavour.
9- Get in the habit of trimming all fat from your meals before cooking. It's a simple step but can help greatly with lowering calories.
10- Check, check, check food labels before you buy. It take a few moment's to do, but you'll be amazed at where all those hidden calories are lurking.
11- Stick to a shopping list when grocery shopping. You'll be less inclined to impulse buy and get the wrong types of food. Also never shop on an empty stomach, it's harder to make the right food choices when you've got a hungry stomach looking for your attention.
12- When shopping head straight to the vegetable and fruit aisle, if you fill your basket there you'll have less room for binge food.
13- Try to make a weekly shopping list and stick to it. The more you return to the grocery store the bigger the chance you'll buy food that you shouldn't.

14- Try varying your food menu eat week. It can be boring eating the same foods over and over again. Try looking online for new recipes or try a new food stuff to wake up your taste buds.

15- Steam your vegetable instead or boiling them, they'll taste nicer and won't lose their nutrition values.

16- Ditch all soft and diet drinks and stick to plain old water. You can add some cordial or a dash of lemon juice to give it some flavour.

17- Have a snack bowl handy for when you're tempted to snack. But have it stocked with nuts, dried fruits and raisins to soothe a sweet tooth.

18- Beware of sampling food as you cook. It's easy to taste as you go and eat more than you should. Also take all unfinished plates straight to the garbage can, if they're left sitting on the sinks draining board you may be inclined to finish off those last pieces of food.

19- Try to stick to more white meat instead or red, and at that only make meat a food choice 2-3 times per week.

20- Never judge a food portion by eye only. If you can't trust yourself or are out of practise, weigh out all your food portions and servings using kitchen scales.

21- Wait no longer than 5 hours between meals, this will help to reduce sugar fluctuations, hunger and keeps your metabolism running smoothly.

22- Keep a food diary at close hand to keep an eye on your eating habits.

23- Try to eat more foods contain fibre, they help to keep you full for longer.

24- Beware of misleading food labels on diet products. Reduced fat means that the item has 25% less fat. Use common sense. If something "normally" contains 300 fat grams, then reduced fat means it still has over 200 grams of fat!

25- If you can't stay away from fatty salad dressings, an easy way to reduce calories is to dip the prongs of your fork in the dressing before you spear the salad. You still get the taste but without the added calories.

26- If you're eating out or even preparing your own, always go for broth types of soup. The clearer the soup, the less calories and fats it has.

27- Take time to both taste your food and chew it. If you eat too fast, your stomach will be full before your brain has time to register it. Think about your food as you taste it, eating should be a pleasant experience and not something that's done quickly before moving on.

28- An easy way to make sure you're never losing out on getting the right nutrition is to vary your foods by colour. One day eat fresh orange and yellow veg like carrots, pumpkin and squash. The next day change to green like lettuce, spinach, cabbage etc.

29- Stick to fruit pies, pumpkin and other fruit pies are lower in calories to pecan pie which has 430 calories per portion compared to 240 calories of pumpkin pie. If you avoid eating the crust you can reduce your calorie count even more.

30- When eating out, make sure to quiz your waiter. Ask plenty of questions, how is the food prepared, how is it cooked. Remember it's your meal so if you want it prepared in a certain way or ingredients left out (within reason) don't be afraid to ask.

31- An easy to reduce calories when eating out is to split a meal between you and friend, or ask for a doggy bag and split your meal before you begin. This way you can save money and calories at the same time.

32- Ditch the chocolate and use cocoa instead when cooking. When cooking 3 tablespoons of cocoa powder can be substituted instead of an ounce of unsweetened chocolate.

33- When making soups and sauces, use evaporated skim milk instead of full fat cream. It has a similar flavour and texture as cream, but with a lower calorie count.

34- Some low fat foods can be a bit bland so why not spic them up. Add herbs like, garlic, basil, onion, oregano and other types of herbs to put some zing in their foods. Spicy foods also have a tendency to curb appetite. People who ate hot peppers ate on average 200 less calories over 3 hours than those that didn't.

THANKS FOR PURCHASING "ESCAPE THAT FAT"

I hope you've enjoyed reading and now have a better game plan to losing weight permanently. I'd really love to read your comments on the book. If you enjoyed this book and found it helpful, please leave a review, this helps me to get this book in front of more new readers and help others.

Why not check out my other book on Sugar Addiction.

UK Amazon Kindle Store http://www.amazon.co.uk/Sugar-Addiction-Beat-Today-ebook/dp/B009A6KBNG

US Amazon Kindle Store http://www.amazon.com/Sugar-Addiction-Beat-Today-ebook/dp/B009A6KBNG

CA Amazon Kindle Store http://www.amazon.ca/Sugar-Addiction-Beat-Today-ebook/dp/B009A6KBNG